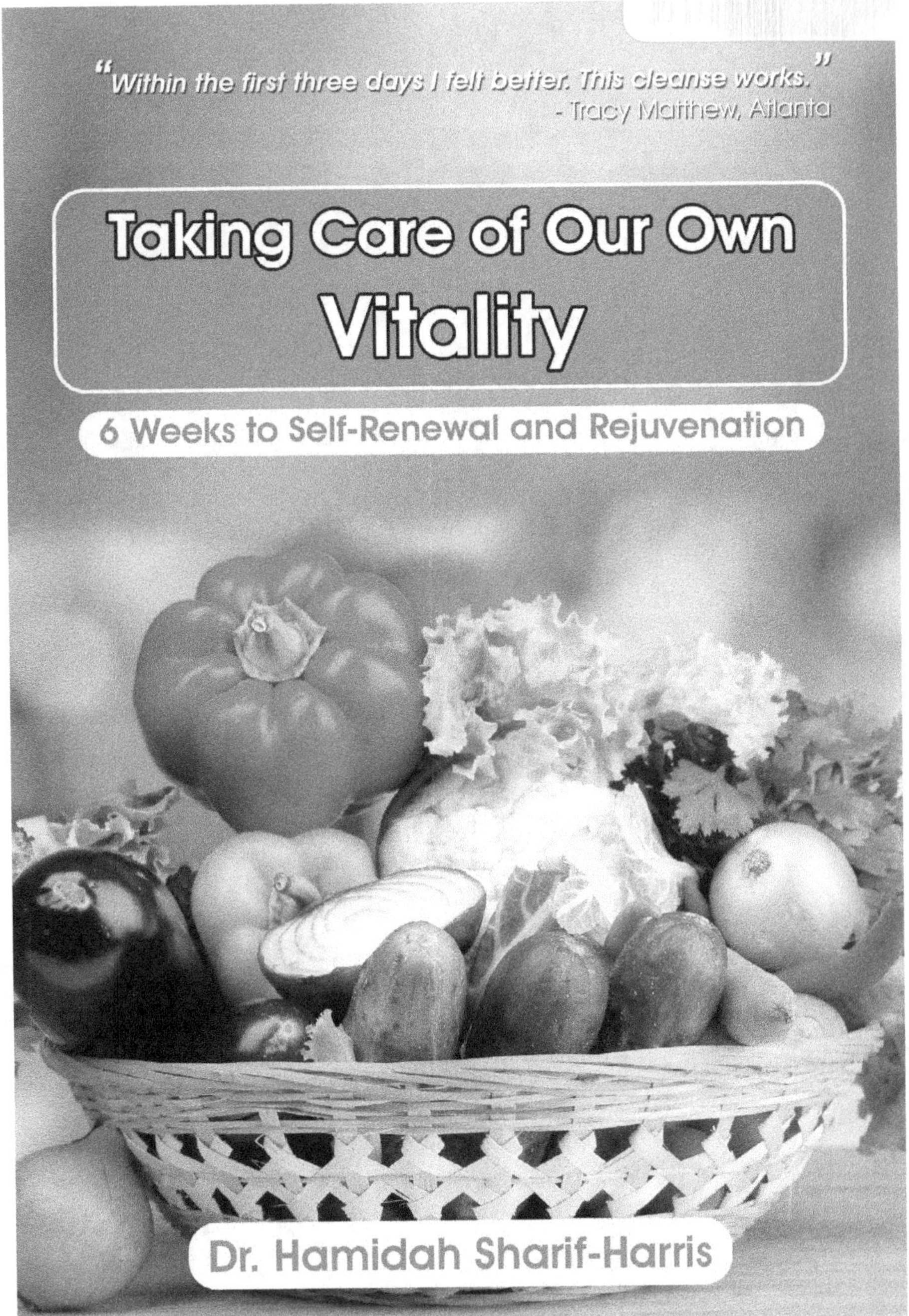

I0412078

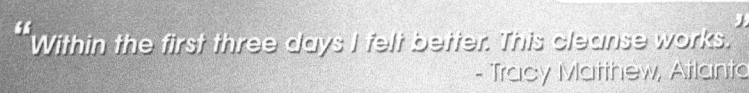

"Within the first three days I felt better. This cleanse works."
- Tracy Matthew, Atlanta

Taking Care of Our Own
Vitality

6 Weeks to Self-Renewal and Rejuvenation

Dr. Hamidah Sharif-Harris

Thrive Well Company, LLC

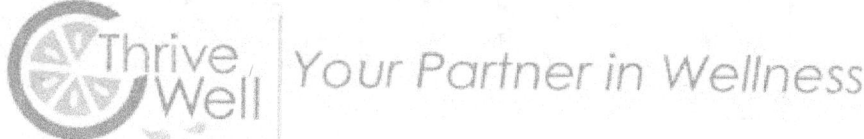

2146 Roswell Road, Suite 108-622, Marietta, GA 30062

www.thrivewellcompany.com

The information contained in this book is not intended to be used to diagnose or prescribe in any way. This book is not meant to take the place of advice from a qualified health care practitioner.

The Guided Herbal Detoxification Program

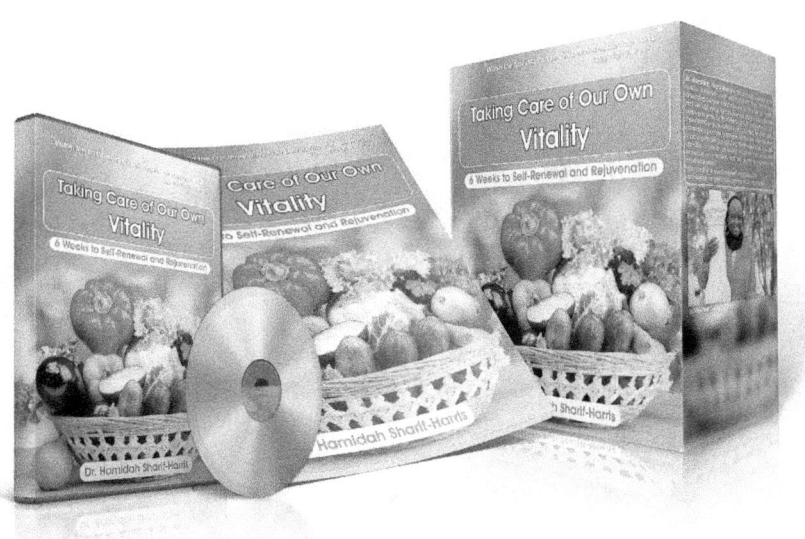

- *6 Week Herbal Detoxification Guidebook*

- *Success Resource Kit*

- *Complete Herbal and Supplement Kit*

- *6 Weekly Guided Sessions with Dr. Sharif-Harris*

- *Access to online VIP Client Success Portal*

Enroll at www.drhamidahsharif.com

In the Name of God, the Most Gracious, the Most Merciful

Many thanks!

I would like to offer my deepest thanks to the Creator who has carried me on a journey through challenge and triumph for my entire life. I am forever grateful to my supportive husband Ishmael, whose selflessness and support of my goals and dreams is unyielding. To my sweet and loving children, Naelah and Qadar who inspire me to be better, do better, and live better. To my mother for her sacrifices and wisdom and to my siblings, whose spirits helped craft me into the faithful woman I have become. God bless all of you.

Please Read.

Dr. Sharif-Harris is a trained health educator and herbalist. She is not a licensed medical doctor and does not diagnose or treat conditions. This information is not a substitute for seeking advice from a medical doctor. Dr. Sharif-Harris will educate and guide you to understand the causes of your conditions and empower you with information to help your body heal itself. The statements about the herbal formulas in this book have not been evaluated by the Food & Drug Administration. These products are not intended to diagnose, treat, cure or prevent disease.

About the Author

Dr. Sharif-Harris provides individualized health education services for clients seeking to better understand their health, achieve optimal wellness, establish healthier lifestyles, promote self-healing, and avoid chronic disease using natural healing therapies. Dr. Sharif-Harris is also an advocate of family-owned organic farming using sustainable development practices. She is a permaculturist and organic gardener for her family's homestead and gardening operations in Georgia.

Dr. Hamidah S. Sharif-Harris was born and raised in Harlem, New York City as one of six children with both of her parents having lived with life-threatening illnesses. Her father was diagnosed with HIV in 1986 and while he has advanced to AIDS twice, he continues to survive the infection today. Her mother was diagnosed with breast cancer at 45 years old which later spread to her thyroid and lungs, however she is a 20 year survivor as well. In 2012, her long-time best friend and sister-in-law, at age 37 and a few months shy of her Ph. D graduation, died unexpectedly while in her sleep after suffering for three years with painful intrauterine fibroids. For the past 20 years, Dr. Sharif-Harris has struggled herself with maintaining a healthy weight and adhering to the demands of life, family, work, and a living a healthy lifestyle. For Dr. Sharif-Harris, promoting health and wellness is not just business, it is personal.

Dr. Sharif-Harris began her career in Harlem, New York as a community health educator and for the past 15 years, she has worked as a Health Education Specialist and wellness consultant for corporations, schools, small businesses and community programs. During her tenure, she also served as Assistant Professor of Health Education and Program Coordinator for Health Education at the University System of Maryland's Coppin State University. In 2008, Dr. Sharif-Harris launched the Thrive Well Company which works with government employees to develop and maintain healthier lifestyle habits.

Dr. Sharif-Harris received several graduate degrees in health education and her Doctorate in Health & Behavior Studies from Columbia University in the City of New York and a Bachelor of Arts in Social Sciences from Adelphi University in New York. Upon moving to Georgia, Dr. Sharif-Harris received Certification in Herbalism from the prestigious School of Natural Healing founded by Dr. John R. Christopher. In addition, Dr. Sharif-Harris has received numerous certifications and advanced diplomas in health and wellness and natural healing therapies.

Dedication

How long does a friendship last? I had one best friend: a soul sister, sister friend, sister-in-law, Soror, all rolled into one. It was the best! And when God decided it was her time to return, she left with him. It's been pretty hard making sense of my new life without a sidekick, another sister perspective on life's obstacles, but so far I have made it through. Yesterday was my birthday and I had a fabulous day, fully blessed. I did think about her in the morning when I discovered a wonderful surprise of flowers and balloons from my husband. But the fast pace of the rest of the day's events occupied most of my thoughts. Lo and behold, I went to sleep last night and my BFF came to visit me in my dreams. Words cannot describe how good it felt to be with my best friend again. We danced and partied, and it felt so real. So how long does a friendship last? I guess if it's real, Forever! I love you Shaquana Anderson. Thank you for twenty years of sisterhood and friendship. This book is dedicated to you!

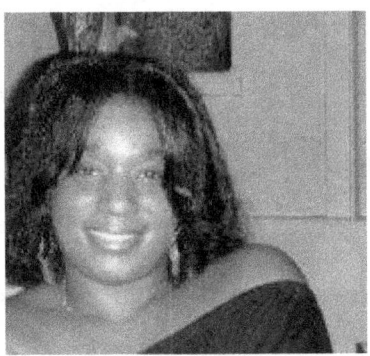

About this program

This program is based on Dr. Christopher's Extended Herbal Cleanse which has been used for over 50 years in the United States and abroad. Dr. Christopher's Cleanse uses whole herbs and organic foods to purify the body so it can be healed naturally. If you are overweight, this program will take you down to your normal body weight; and if you are underweight, it will bring you up to normal. The purpose of the entire program is to eliminate mucus, congestion, toxins including heavy metals so your body is able to function in the way God intended. After you have completed this cleanse, continue eating mucus-less foods and you will be delighted at how amazing you will look and feel.

How to Use this Book

1. Answer the questions about your experiences in the section provided.

2. Note reactions to herbs or foods in the weekly log.

3. Weigh yourself twice only. Once before you begin, and again after you have completed the 6 Week Cleanse.

Table of Contents

Chapter 1: A New Beginning

"Sick and Tired of Being Sick and Tired"

-Fannie Lou Hamer

My Story

I am a workaholic. I work to forget pain. I work to overcome frustration. I work to escape the challenges of family life. I work to excuse myself from crying and breaking down. I work to distract myself from the necessary self-work that I need to do. Of course, every workaholic needs fuel; my fuel was coffee. I consumed 3 to 5 cups of coffee everyday for years. After my best friend passed away, I began to take a hard long look at myself spiritually and physically. A year after losing Shaquana, I received news that my childhood friend Sheryl was killed by her boyfriend. I reflected on the choices Sheryl and I made as adolescents and how those choice impacted my adulthood. Before I could recover from her loss, I learned a close friend from high school had also died from breast cancer. In just three short years, I lost three sister-friends, all young, all beautiful, all with long lives still left to live.

My time for excuses was finished. I decided it was time to do the hard work to find the peace I knew the Creator wanted me to have. Frustrated with my spiritual and physical state, I began reading my Holy book and digging deeper into the lesson the Creator wanted me to learn. It was during this time, that I began to return to my interest in herbs and natural healing.

This was a time in my life when I was feeling exhausted, sluggish, bloated, and quite frankly, old and worn out. Each of my bodily systems felt contaminated and toxic. At 39 years old, I felt more like a 70 year old without an ounce of energy.

I suffered from migraines, painful menstrual cramps, lower backache, dry skin, and chronic obesity. I reached the point where I understood what Fannie Lou Hamer meant when she said she was "sick and tired, of being sick and tired."

A change needed to happen immediately. I decided to enroll in the Family Herbalist course at the School of Natural Healing to get a holistic understanding of how to properly cleanse my body.

When I finished the program, I ordered the Herbal Cleansing Kit and started on the first phase of the program. Within two weeks, my face lost its puffiness, my skin glowed, and the migraines disappeared. When I finished the 6 week regimen, I had shed 15 pounds and was relieved of all the ailments I suffered from for years. This program did not just put me on the path to better physical health, it also keeps my spirit connected to the Creator by focusing on organically-grown fruits, vegetables, whole grains and nuts. My mind has been reconnected to my body and my spirit.

" And God said, Behold, I have given you every herb bearing seed, which is upon the face of all the earth, and every tree, in the which is the fruit of a tree yielding seed; to you it shall be for meat. " - Holy Torah, Genesis 1:29

After completing my initial cleanse, I realized that there were many people who are in the same spiritual and physical place that I was and needed a little help. I decided to document the process I used for my own renewal. This cleansing program is the final product. I have worked with family and friends to help them through this process with awesome results. This will be a life-altering journey that will help you reclaim the youthfulness and vitality that you may have been missing.

This book is titled *Taking Care of Our Own Vitality* because many of us have been waiting for outside intervention (i.e. money, a mate, etc.) to come and fix our problems. We have been given the power to feed, care, heal, and provide for ourselves by the Creator. It's time we take full ownership of that power, starting today.

"For the Spirit that God has given us does not make us timid; instead, his Spirit fills us with power, love, and self-control." Holy Bible, 2 Timothy 1:7

Program Options

I am here. You do not have to take this journey on your own. There are two options for this program.

- You can choose to follow the instructions in this book and purchase the complete herbal cleansing kit online at **drhamidahsharif.com.**

- You can also choose to enroll in my Guided Detox Program utilizing the 6-Week Cleansing Program which includes the cost of the herbal kit and weekly phone consultations with Dr. Sharif. You can enroll online at **drhamidahsharif.com**

You are free to choose whichever method works best for you. I pray you are able to complete your 6-Week Cleanse with ease and that your results are magnificent. Let's begin....

Chapter 2: The Preparatory Fast

"O ye who believe! Fasting is prescribed for you, as it was prescribed for those before you, so that you may become righteous. "

— *Holy Qu'ran, Baqarah 2:183*

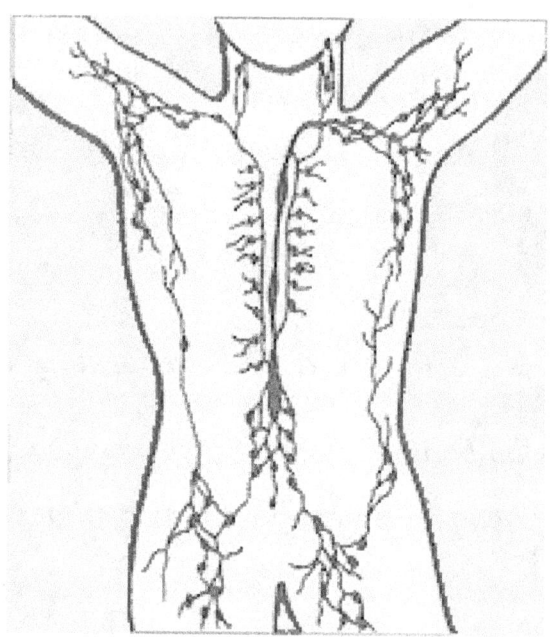

The purpose of this fast is to flush the lymphatic system of toxins and replace the toxic lymph with fresh juices. This fast will draw the toxins from the intestines and every part of the body into the lower bowel for elimination. You can complete this fast for one, two, or three days depending on ability. For some people, three days is very difficult. If you cannot complete three days start with one day and then move to the next phase of the Cleansing program. After the fast up to gallons of toxin lymph will have been eliminated from the body and will have been replaced by three gallons of juices. This will result in speeding up the re-alkalizing of the system. If there is a jaundice condition, Dr. Christopher's Liver Gall Bladder Formula should be used three times a day as well. Be prepared to spend the entire day of fasting at home or near a bathroom.

Supplies needed:

- Steam distilled water (one gallon per day)

- herbal teas*

- organic prune juice*

- your choice of organic fruit juice and the same organic fruit in whole form (apple, carrot, grape, orange, etc.) You must select one type of juice for the entire fast.

- extra virgin olive oil*

*These items are included in the Herbal Supplement Kit.

Your Body During the Fast

Many people experience a range of reactions during the preparatory fast. These reactions include coughing, mucus, congestion, nausea, body aches, etc. Your body will begin cleansing itself during this fasting period and depending upon the areas of your body that are the most congested is where you will notice the most reaction. This is NORMAL. You will also likely feel a bit less energetic as your body becomes accustomed to the loss of its food addictions (i.e. sugar, bread, coffee, soft drinks, dairy, etc.). As you begin the 6 Week Cleanse, your body will quickly recover and you will realize you have more energy than usual. Note that you will continue to have adverse reactions periodically during the 6 Week Cleanse. Sometimes it will feel as though you are ill; however, you will simply be purging the toxins and accumulation of waste in your bodily systems. In addition, you will move your bowels often during the fast. Your bowels will mostly consist of water and mucus. This is NORMAL. You may find comfort in applying a light coat of petroleum jelly to the outer skin of your rectum. Remember, this will only last between one and three days. Trust me, it's worth it!

How to Know If Something Is Wrong

If you experience severe stomach cramping, heart palpitations, elevated blood pressure, fainting, or any other significant health condition during this cleanse, discontinue taking the herbal supplements and seek advice from an herbalist or a trusted health care professional.

These conditions are not side effects of the herbal supplements. Your body may be experiencing a new and significant health condition, which may need immediate attention.

Schedule

Morning

- Drink several cups of herbal tea with honey (or agave) until 10:00 am
- At 10:00 am, drink 16 ounces of organic prune juice
- Within 30 minutes, drink 8 ounces of your chosen fruit juice (Do not gulp this juice. Instead chew it throughout your mouth to mix it well with your saliva).
- 11:00 am Follow the juice with 8 ounces of distilled water
- 11:30 am Drink 8 ounces of fruit juice
- 12:00 pm Follow the juice with 8 ounces of distilled water

Afternoon

- 12:30 pm Take one tablespoon of olive oil by mouth; Drink 8 ounces of fruit juice
- 1:00pm to 6:00pm Repeat alternating the juice with the distilled water
- Eat one or two pieces of fruit (if you are hungry)

Evening

- 6:00 pm Take another tablespoon of olive oil by mouth
- Take two capsules of Lower Bowel Formula
- Continue with alternating the juice with the distilled water
- Eat one or two pieces of fruit (if you are hungry)

Bedtime

- 10:00 pm Take your last 8 ounces of distilled water
- Take another tablespoon of olive oil by mouth

	PREPARATORY FAST 1-3 DAYS		
	DAY 1	**DAY 2**	**DAY 3**
MORNING	Wake – 10:00am ☐ Drink several cups of herbal tea w/honey or agave ☐ 2 capsules **Lower Bowel formula** 10:00am ☐ 16oz of prune juice 10:30am ☐ 8oz of fruit juice (don't gulp, chew thru mouth to mix w/saliva) 11:00am ☐ 8oz distilled water 11:30am ☐ 8oz fruit juice 12:00pm ☐ 8oz distilled water	Wake – 10:00am ☐ Drink several cups of herbal tea w/honey or agave ☐ 2 capsules **Lower Bowel formula** 10:00am ☐ 16oz of prune juice 10:30am ☐ 8oz of fruit juice (don't gulp, chew thru mouth to mix w/saliva) 11:00am ☐ 8oz distilled water 11:30am ☐ 8oz fruit juice 12:00pm ☐ 8oz distilled water	Wake – 10:00am ☐ Drink several cups of herbal tea w/honey or agave ☐ 2 capsules **Lower Bowel formula** 10:00am ☐ 16oz of prune juice 10:30am ☐ 8oz of fruit juice (don't gulp, chew thru mouth to mix w/saliva) 11:00am ☐ 8oz distilled water 11:30am ☐ 8oz fruit juice 12:00pm ☐ 8oz distilled water
AFTERNOON	12:00pm ☐ 2 capsules **Lower Bowel Formula** 12:30pm ☐ 1 tbsp olive oil ☐ 8oz fruit juice 1:00pm – 6:00pm ☐ Repeat alternating 8oz distilled water with 8oz fruit juice *1-2 pieces of fruit if hungry	12:00pm ☐ 2 capsules **Lower Bowel Formula** 12:30pm ☐ 1 tbsp olive oil ☐ 8oz fruit juice 1:00pm – 6:00pm ☐ Repeat alternating 8oz distilled water with 8oz fruit juice *1-2 pieces of fruit if hungry	12:00pm ☐ 2 capsules **Lower Bowel Formula** 12:30pm ☐ 1 tbsp olive oil ☐ 8oz fruit juice 1:00pm – 6:00pm ☐ Repeat alternating 8oz distilled water with 8oz fruit juice *1-2 pieces of fruit if hungry
EVENING	6:00pm – 10:00pm ☐ 2 capsules **Lower Bowel formula** ☐ Repeat alternating 8oz fruit juice with 8oz distilled water	6:00pm – 10:00pm ☐ 2 capsules **Lower Bowel formula** ☐ Repeat alternating 8oz fruit juice with 8oz distilled water	6:00pm – 10:00pm ☐ 2 capsules **Lower Bowel formula** ☐ Repeat alternating 8oz fruit juice with 8oz distilled water
BEDTIME	10:00pm 8oz distilled water 1 tbsp olive oil	10:00pm 8oz distilled water 1 tbsp olive oil	10:00pm 8oz distilled water 1 tbsp olive oil

Chapter 3: Getting Ready

"O ye who believe! Persevere in patience and constancy;

- Holy Qu'ran, Al-Imran 3:200

I suggest getting prepared for this cleanse with deep meditation or prayer. While it is a physical experience, I believe the spirit must also be ready to deal with the challenges, fears and frustrations that come with a lifestyle change. You can help prepare yourself by spending quiet time alone in the early morning hours and the late evening hours thinking about who you are and who you would like to become. The process of healing takes time and patience. Take your time and don't rush yourself. If you make a mistake or eat something that is not helpful to help your body maintain the efficiency God intended, it's okay. Negative self-talk will not help in your healing process. Be gentle with yourself.

Preparing to Cleanse

When you are dealing with long standing health problems, you cannot expect to totally cleanse the body with one three day cleansing routines. Therefore, to rid the body of chronic conditions or to help stop their occurrence, an extended herbal cleanse is an excellent path to follow. Be sure to follow these guidelines and you will have success.

1. Take the following herbal extracts as directed until the formulas are gone.

2. Tailor this program to fit your individual body's needs.

3. Drink a minimum of 8 to 16 glasses of distilled water each day between meals.

4. Avoid mucus promoting foods such as dairy products and fatty red meats as much as possible.

5. Increase your intake of fresh vegetables, grains, seeds, and nuts.

6. If you have any questions or concerns about beginning this intensive cleansing program we recommend that you consult with your health practitioner.

Supplies Needed:

These are provided in the Herbal Supplement Kit

- Steam distilled water

- organic cayenne pepper*

- organic raw honey*

- organic apple cider vinegar with the mother*

- unsulphured molasses*

- wheat germ oil*

- herbal teas

Dr. Christopher's Herbal Formulas:**

- Lower Bowel Formula

- Liver and Gallbladder Formula

- Kidney Formula

- Blood Stream Formula

*Provided in the Complete Herbal and Supplement Kit

**Herbal formulas needed are available in capsules and extract.

You can purchase the Complete 6-Week Herbal Cleansing Kit (including the supplies) at drhamidahsharif.com. Alternatively, you can visit your local health food store and purchase each of the herbs in the formulas, and drink the formulas as a brewed tea.

Implement the healing practices of this program for 6 days, followed by 1 full day's rest (do not take any herbal formulas or supplements). It may be helpful for you to also allow one day to enjoy one or two of your favorite foods that is not on the recommended food list. Remember, all things in moderation.

The Lower Bowel Formula contains golden seal which is a very bitter herb. Many people find it easier to take it in capsule form. However, if you would like to take the liquid, add 2 droppersful to 8 ounces of orange juice and the taste will not be offensive.

Tips and Suggestions:

- Eat as many portions of the foods on this list as you like. Snacking on healthy foods will not harm your detoxification progress.

- It is best to make your own condiments using fresh herbs, peppers, olive oil and apple cider vinegar.
- Simplify the administration of the extracts by mixing the dosages into one 8 oz. cup of orange juice or other acidic fruit juice. The acidity will equalize the bitterness of the formulas.
- Do not resist the urge to urinate or defecate. Allow your body to eliminate naturally.

Chapter 4: The Lower Bowel

"Well over 90% of all disease comes from an unclean body whose sewer is backed up"

- Dr. John R. Christopher

Week 1 and 2

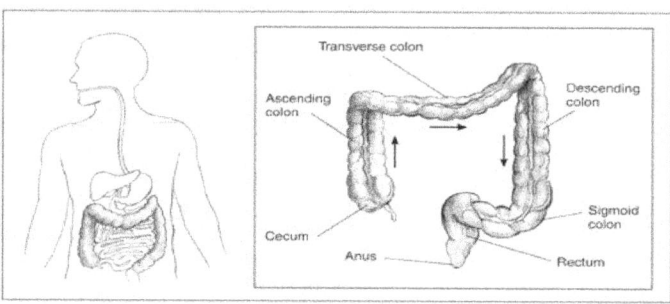

Our colon is a neglected organ. It is responsible for removing all the toxic waste and material from our bodies and sending it out of our bodies. The foods we eat on the average American diet have significantly impaired its functioning. Many of the unwholesome foods we eat create mucus that adheres to our intestinal walls. The mucus becomes like a paste and forms layers around the intestinal walls. As we continue to eat mucus filled foods, we add additional layers of mucus paste and the muscular and absorptive tissues become covered and dysfunctional. Finally, once the fecal layers have become hardened and thicker, only a small hole remains for fecal passage. Many people believe they have regular bowel movements; however, most Americans are severely constipated. The fecal matter stuck inside our intestinal walls prevents the food we are eating from being assimilated by the body. In fact, according to Dr. Christopher, only 10% of what we eat is actually assimilated to feed our body cells. The general rule is one bowel movement per meal. Therefore, if you are not having a bowel movement after every meal, you are very likely constipated.

Dr. Christopher's Lower Bowel Formula:

This is one of Dr. Christopher's most famous and popular formulas. One of the most important and beneficial factors of this formula is how it stimulates peristaltic action within the lower bowel and the whole body. This formula re-builds the tissues of the colon and strengthens the intestinal muscles. A clear and flowing lower bowel can avoid many health conditions.

Ingredients: barberry, cascara sagrada, cayenne, ginger, lobelia, red raspberry, turkey rhubarb, fennel, golden seal. You can purchase these herbal plants and brew this formula as a tea. Alternatively, you can use the prepared capsules or tincture in the Herbal Cleansing Program Kit.

Dosage: 2 capsules, 3 times per day. (If you do not move bowels after each meal increase to 3 capsules/3 times a day or 4 capsules/3 times a day. If you are severely constipated, please consult your herbalist or health care professional for further instructions. Alternatively, you can drink one cup of tea with each meal.

Warning: Do not use this product when abdominal pain, nausea or vomiting are present. Rectal bleeding or failure to have a bowel movement after use of laxative may indicate a serious problem. Discontinue use and consult with your health care professional.

Week 1 and Week 2

Morning:

- Upon rising, drink one or more cups of distilled water.

- Drink one cup of fresh juices and/or one cup of herbal tea

- Eat a breakfast of your choice using foods on the food list

- Take a dose of the Lower Bowel Formula prior to your meal

- Mix one tablespoon of apple cider vinegar and honey and take by mouth

- Take one teaspoon each of molasses and wheat germ oil

- Drink one cup of distilled water each hour of the day while awake

Afternoon

- Eat a lunch of your choice using the foods on the food list

- Take another dose of Lower Bowel Formula prior to your meal

- Take another tablespoon of apple cider vinegar and honey by mouth

- Take one teaspoon each of molasses and wheat germ oil

- Continue drinking distilled water every hour

Evening

- Eat a dinner of your choice using the foods on the food list

- Take another dose of the Lower Bowel Formula prior to your meal

- Take another tablespoon of apple cider vinegar and honey by mouth

- Take one teaspoon each of molasses and wheat germ oil

- Continue drinking distilled water every hour

What physical changes did you notice after completing the first two weeks?

_____

_____

_____

_____

_____

What changes in mood or attitude have you discovered after completing the first two weeks?

_____

_____

_____

_____

_____

List any challenges you faced with adhering to the herbal regimen or the mucus-less eating plan.

_____

_____

_____

_____

_____

Brainstorm some ideas to counteract these challenges

_____

_____

_____

_____

_____

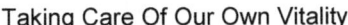

Chapter 5: Liver and Gallbladder

Our Personal Bodyguard

Week 3

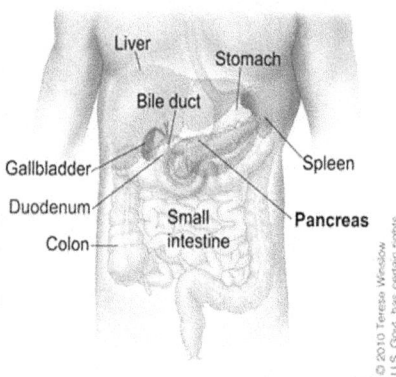

The liver has numerous functions in the body. One of its main jobs is to filter the blood as it travels throughout the circulatory system. When the liver is not functioning many conditions may result including acne, eczema, hormonal problems, manic depression, anxiety, depression, loss of libido, constipation, cholemia, indigestion, sluggishness, fatigue, upset stomach, chills, vomiting, and fever.

Dr. Christopher's Liver and Gallbladder Formula:

The Liver and Gall bladder formula supports the proper function of both the liver and gall bladder and helps rebuild and cleanse these organs. Ingredients: barberry, wild yam, cramp bark, fennel, ginger, catnip, and peppermint.

Dosage: 15 to 30 drops prior to each meal or 2 capsules three times a day or one cup of tea with each meal.

Week 3

Morning:

- Upon rising, drink one or more cups of distilled water.

- Drink one cup of fresh juices and/or one cup of herbal tea

- Take a dose of Liver and Gall bladder Formula prior to your breakfast

- Eat a breakfast of your choice using foods on the food list

- Take a dose of Lower Bowel Formula prior to your meal

- Mix one tablespoon of apple cider vinegar and honey and take by mouth*

- Take one teaspoon each of molasses and wheat germ oil*

- Drink one cup of distilled water each hour of the day while awake

Afternoon

- Take another dose of the Liver and Gall bladder Formula prior to your lunch

- Eat a lunch of your choice using the foods on the food list

- Take another dose of Lower Bowel Formula

- Take another tablespoon of apple cider vinegar and honey by mouth

- Take one teaspoon each of molasses and wheat germ oil

- Continue drinking distilled water every hour

Evening

- Take another dose of the Liver and Gall bladder Formula prior to your meal

- Eat a dinner of your choice using the foods on the food list

- Take another dose of the Lower Bowel Formula prior to your meal

- Take another tablespoon of apple cider vinegar and honey by mouth

- Take one teaspoon each of molasses and wheat germ oil

- Continue drinking distilled water every hour

What physical changes did you notice after completing the first three weeks?

_____

_____

_____

_____

_____

What changes in mood or attitude have you discovered after completing the first three weeks?

_____

_____

_____

_____

_____

List any challenges you faced with adhering to the herbal regimen or the mucus-less eating plan.

_____

_____

_____

_____

_____

Brainstorm some ideas to counteract these challenges.

_____

_____

_____

_____

_____

Chapter 6: The Kidney and Bladder

Our Subway System

Week 4

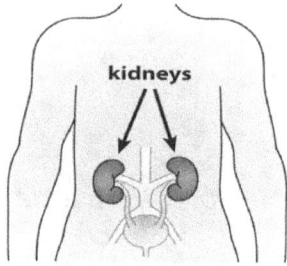

Nearly 80% of the body is liquid, and most of the fluid must be pumped and filtered through the urinary system. Unfortunately, we do not take the best care of this important organ. Its job includes circulating fluids. Many of the fluids that we have gotten the most accustomed to ingesting cause irritation and clogging. These words of these include tea, coffee, soft drinks, hard water, alcohol, etc. Often, the result is malfunctioning kidneys, kidney stones, and lower back pain.

Dr. Christopher's Kidney Formula: This formula is a specific for the kidneys. Over the years we have used a formula of herbs with people who have been afraid to be out in public because of lack of control over the urinary tract and unknowingly voiding urine. After using this formula, many people have found relief from this condition and are living normal lives again. This formula provides specific nutrition for the kidneys and bladder, cleans out deposits, and strengthens the urinary tract walls and muscles. It is also useful for urinary incontinence. Ingredients: Juniper Berry, Parsley Root, Uva Ursi Leaf, Marshmallow Root, Lobelia Herb, Ginger Root & Goldenseal Root.

Dosage: 15 to 30 drops prior to each meal or 2 capsules three times a day or one cup of tea with each meal.

Warning: Do not use during pregnancy or while nursing except as directed by your health care professional.

Morning:

- Upon rising, drink one or more cups of distilled water.

- Drink one cup of fresh juices and/or one cup of herbal tea

- Eat a breakfast of your choice using foods on the food list

- Take a dose of the Lower Bowel Formula prior to your meal

- Take a dose of the Liver & Gall bladder Formula prior to your meal

- Take a dose of the Kidney Formula prior to your meal

- Mix one tablespoon of apple cider vinegar and honey and take by mouth*

- Take one teaspoon each of molasses and wheat germ oil*

- Drink one cup of distilled water each hour of the day while awake

Afternoon

- Eat a lunch of your choice using the foods on the food list

- Take another dose of Lower Bowel Formula prior to your meal

- Take another dose of the Liver & Gall bladder Formula

- Take another dose of the Kidney Formula prior to your meal

- Take another tablespoon of apple cider vinegar and honey by mouth

- Take one teaspoon each of molasses and wheat germ oil

- Continue drinking distilled water every hour

Evening

- Eat a dinner of your choice using the foods on the food list

- Take another dose of the Lower Bowel Formula prior to your meal

- Take another dose of the Liver & Gall bladder Formula prior to your meal

- Take another dose of the Kidney Formula prior to your meal

- Take another tablespoon of apple cider vinegar and honey by mouth

- Take one teaspoon each of molasses and wheat germ oil

- Continue drinking distilled water every hour

What physical changes did you notice after completing the first four weeks?

_____

_____

_____

_____

_____

What changes in mood or attitude have you discovered after completing the first four weeks?

_____

_____

_____

_____

_____

List any challenges you faced with adhering to the herbal regimen or the mucus-less eating plan.

_____

_____

_____

_____

Brainstorm some ideas to counteract these challenges.

_____

_____

_____

_____

_____

_____

Chapter 7: The Blood

Our Internal Transportation System

Week 5 and 6

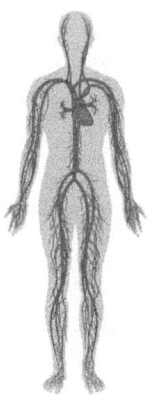

Dr. Christopher's Blood Stream Formula: This formula helps promote a healthy and clean blood stream. The blood stream is life itself, and it is our job to keep it clean and pure so that we can have a good circulatory system for delivering food to the body properly and to carry off the waste materials.

This herbal blood re-builder is made up of herbs that are cleansers and astringents. Other herbs aid in removing cholesterol, killing infection, and building elasticity in the veins and strengthening the vein and artery walls. This extract is in a base of pure vegetable glycerin. This aid is designed to help cleanse the blood down to the cellular level. It also aids in removing cholesterol, builds elasticity and strength in veins and artery walls. This formula also contains herbs that are potent infection fighters. Ingredients: red clover, chaparral, licorice, poke root, peach bark, Oregon grape, stillingia, cascara sagrada, sarsaparilla, prickly ash, and burdock.

Dosage: 5 to 15 drops prior to each meal or 2 capsules three times a day or One cup of tea with each meal.

Week 5 and Week 6

Morning:

- Upon rising, drink one or more cups of distilled water.

- Drink one cup of fresh juices and/or one cup of herbal tea

- Eat a breakfast of your choice using foods on the food list

- Take dose of the Lower Bowel Formula prior to your meal

- Take dose of the Liver & Gall bladder Formula prior to your meal

- Take dose of the Kidney Formula prior to your meal

- Take a dose before each meal of the Blood Stream Formula

- Mix one tablespoon of apple cider vinegar and honey and take by mouth*

- Take one teaspoon each of molasses and wheat germ oil*

- Drink one cup of distilled water each hour of the day while awake

Afternoon

- Eat a lunch of your choice using the foods on the food list

- Take another dose of Lower Bowel Formula prior to your meal

- Take a dose of Liver & Gall bladder Formula prior to your meal

- Take a dose of the Kidney Formula prior to your meal

- Take a dose of the Blood Stream Formula prior to your meal

- Take another tablespoon of apple cider vinegar and honey by mouth

- Take one teaspoon each of molasses and wheat germ oil

- Continue drinking distilled water every hour

Evening

- Eat a dinner of your choice using the foods on the food list

- Take another dose of the Lower Bowel Formula prior to each meal

- Take another dose of the Liver & Gall bladder Formula prior to each meal

- Take another dose of the Kidney Formula prior to your meal

- Take another dose of the Blood Stream Formula prior to your meal

- Take another tablespoon of apple cider vinegar and honey by mouth

- Take one teaspoon each of molasses and wheat germ oil

- Continue drinking distilled water every hour

What physical changes did you notice after completing week 5 and 6?

_____

_____

_____

_____

_____

What changes in mood or attitude have you discovered after completing week 5 and 6?

_____

_____

_____

_____

List any challenges you faced with adhering to the herbal regimen or the mucus-less eating plan.

_____

_____

_____

_____

Brainstorm some ideas to counteract these challenges.

_____

_____

_____

_____

Chapter 8: Food Lists

Focus on increasing your servings of healthful mucusless foods instead of reducing the mucus-filled foods.

Food Lists

You can create many delicious meals using these mucusless foods. Please eat as many as you like, as often as you would like. You will be satisfied and healing your own body.

ACID-BINDING, NON-MUCUS-FORMING,

OR MUCUSLESS (MUCUS-FREE) FOODS

GREEN LEAF VEGETABLES (MUCUSLESS)

Arugula

Bok Choi

Cabbage

Collard

Dandelion Leaf

Kale

Leafy Herbs (Basil, Parsley, Cilantro, Rosemary, Thyme, etc.)

Lettuce (Green, Red, Romaine, Boston Bibb, Iceberg)

Mustard

Spinach

Swiss chard

Turnip

Watercress

RAW VEGETABLES/ROOT, STEM, FRUIT
(ALL OR RELATIVELY STARCHLESS/MUCUSLESS)

Asparagus

Black Radish, with skin

Broccoli

Brussels Sprouts

Celery

Cucumbers

Dandelion

Dill

Endives

Green Onions

Horse Radish, with skin

Leeks

Onions

Peppers (Green, Red, Yellow, or Orange)

Red Beets

Red Cabbage

Rhubarb

Sea Vegetables

Sprouts (Alfalfa, Brassica, Green-Leaf, Radish)

Sugar Beets

Tomatoes

Young Radish

Zucchini

BAKED VEGETABLES ROOT, STEM, FRUIT
(ALL OR RELATIVELY STARCHLESS/MUCUSLESS)

Acorn Squash (Baked)

Asparagus

Broccoli (Baked or Steamed)

Brussels Sprouts (Steamed)

Butternut Squash (Baked)

Carrots (Steamed)

Cauliflower (Steamed or Baked)

Green Peas (Steamed)

Peppers (Green, Red, Yellow, or Orange)

Peppers (Green, Red, Yellow, or Orange)

Pumpkins (Baked or Steamed)

Spaghetti Squash (Baked)

Sweet Potato (Baked)

Zucchini (Steamed or Baked)

RIPE FRUITS (MUCUSLESS)

Apples

Apricots

Banana

Black Cherries

Blackberries

Blood Orange

Cantaloupe

Cherries

Grapefruit

Grapes

Honeybell Tangelos

Honeydew

Lemons

Mandarin

Mangos

Nectarine

Oranges

Papaya

Peaches

Pears

Pineapple

Plums

Pomegranates

Prunes

Raisins

Raspberries

Sour Cherries

Strawberries

Sweet Cherries

Sweet Cherries

Tangerines

Tangerines

Watermelon

DRIED OR BAKED FRUITS (MUCUSLESS)

Apples

Apricots

Bananas

Blueberries

Cherries

Cranberries

Currants

Currants, (Dried)

Dates

Dates, (Dried)

Figs

Figs (Dried)

Grapes/raisins

Kiwi

Mango

Peaches

Pears

Pineapple

Plums/prunes

Strawberries

100% FRUIT JELLIES, SYRUPS, AND HONEY

Agave Nectar

Coconut Water

Fruit Jellies (no sugar added)

Maple Syrup (100%, no preservatives)

Molasses (no preservatives)

Honey (bee)

ENJOY THESE PROTEINS

Lean organic halal/kosher chicken

Lean grass-fed halal/kosher beef (no more than 1-2 times per week)

Plenty of wild salmon (not farm-raised)

Other light fish (no more than 1-2 times per week)

Avoid these foods as they contain A LOT of mucus

Eggs

Cheese

Dairy

White sugar/brown sugar

Flour (except brown rice flour)

Breads

Pastas (except whole grain pasta)

Cereals (except whole oatmeal, Steel cut oats preferably)

Chapter 9:

Maintenance

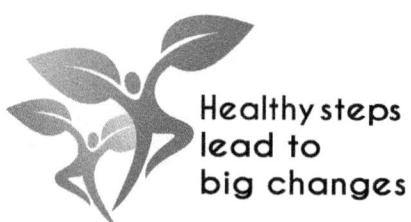

Healthy steps
lead to
big changes

Congratulations! You have completed the first step towards to living a physically and spiritually healthier life. You should be extremely proud of yourself. Now, let's discuss how to keep your momentum going. It is recommended that you take one week of rest after ending your 6 Week Herbal Cleanse. If you did not achieve your optimum state of weight or bodily functioning, then you should repeat the 6 week Cleanse for the next six months, taking one week breaks between each cleanse. In addition to the cleansing herbs, you should also add the following items to your daily regimen. After six months of cleansing, eating mucus-free foods, and exercising, reassess your health status with your herbalist or health care provider for next steps.

Your ability to keep yourself healthy and maintaining your ideal weight will depend on how well you continue to eat mucus-free foods, drink water, and get exercise.

EXERCISE

For steady weight management, exercise daily. The best exercise for cleansing and weight management is the re-bounder. This mini-trampoline moves lymphatic fluid throughout the body and improves cardiovascular endurance.

MAINTENANCE HERBS

Dr. Christopher Metaburn (Official Product Description)

A synergistic blend of whole herbs designed to assist the body in burning calories while controlling the appetite & hunger pains. Maintaining a healthy weight can be hard in our fast food, massive portion sized culture & losing weight can be even tougher. Adding to the difficulty is all the quick fixes & fad diets that tempt & confuse us.

If your weight is a balancing act, then there are plenty of small but powerful changes that will help you achieve lasting weight loss, such as avoiding common dieting pitfalls, develop a healthy plan with enjoyable choices, eating fewer calories than you burn & our best friend exercise. Traditional diets don't tend to work in the long term as most formulas out in the marketplace deplete the body of vital nutrition.

Dr. Christopher's Metaburn Herbal Weight helps to curb appetite & supplies the essential vitamins & minerals needed for proper body function during weight management. Metaburn Herbal Weight Capsule is a complex vitamin of natural biologically active substances of plant origin, which optimizes metabolic processes in the body and helps to normalize weight and enrich the diet with beneficial biologically active substances.

The common therapeutic effects of this formulation include:

• Helps to burn fat more efficiently

• Prevents the deposition of fat in tissues

• Improves skin condition

• Helps to remove toxins from the body

• Optimizes the functioning of the gastrointestinal tract

• Contributes to rapid recovery after different diseases

• Helps to treat chronic fatigue syndrome

• Normalizes blood circulation and the intestinal function

• Normalizes metabolism and helps to burn fat more efficiently

• Enhances the immune defenses

Dr. Christopher's formula is a rich source of herbal vitamins A, C, B1, B2, E, and P. Vitamin P strengthens the walls of blood vessels and contributes to the accumulation of vitamin C. A large iron content allows for the prevention of iron deficiency anemia after prolonged chronic illnesses. The Metaburn formula is formulated with herbs known for their rich content of substances that have the ability to bind toxins and waste products (heavy metals, radioactive elements) and remove them from the body. This plays an important role in the prevention of some intestinal diseases and speeds up blood clotting.

Proprietary Blend: *
Brigham Tea Herb, Red Clover Blossom, Oat straw Herb, Damiana Leaf, Chickweed Herb, Juniper Berry, Catnip Herb, Senna Leaf & Cayenne Pepper.

Take 3 capsules two times a day. Avoid taking this product after 2 pm. as it may interfere with normal sleep patterns. For optimum results take 1 hour before or after meals as to not compete with digestion. Store in a cool, dry place. Keep out of reach of children.

Dr. Christopher Vitalerbs (Official Product Description)

Vitalerbs are a nature-balanced whole food vitamin & mineral supplement for the body. Vitamins & minerals play a key role in boosting the immune system, growth & development, mental aptitude, physical fitness & in supporting the body's systems. Eating a variety of healthy foods is the best way to get all the vitamins & minerals you need each day but many skip meals, diet or do not eat enough items from a particular food category, such as vegetables or fruit. The market is flooded with standardized supplements, which extract leading active ingredients but Dr. Christopher's Vitalerbs is the ultimate whole-food formula, perfectly balanced the way Mother Nature intended with vitamins & minerals.

Proprietary Blend: *
Jurassic Green (Certified Organic Flash-Dried Juice Powder from Alfalfa, Barley & Non-Hybrid Wheat Grass), Dandelion Root, Kelp Plant, Purple Dulse Leaf, Spirulina, Irish Moss, Rose hips, Beet Root, Nutritional Yeast, Cayenne Pepper, Blue Violet Leaf, Oat straw Herb, Carrot & Ginger Root.

Take 2 capsules three times a day or as directed by your Health Care Professional. For optimum results take 1 hour before or after meals as to not compete with digestion. Store in a cool, dry place. Keep out of reach of children.

Other Health Conditions

If you suffer from other health conditions including female menstrual complaints, sluggish thyroid, blood pressure or blood sugar regulation, or hormonal imbalance many of these issues will relieve themselves during the cleanse. However, if you are still experiencing some of the effects of these symptoms, it would be beneficial for you to supplement your herbal regimen with additional herbs that can target the root causes of those illnesses more specifically. Please visit www.drhamidahsharif.com for more information on these herbal supplements.

RESOURCES

School of Natural Healing

www.snh.cc

Dr. Hamidah Sharif-Harris

www.drhamidahsharif.com

Dr. Christopher's Herbal Education

www.herballegacy.com

Christopher Publications

www.christopherpublications.com

A Healthier You Radio

http://www.ahealthieryouradio.com/

Notes